Paediatric  an Examination

Ian A. Laing
MA, MD, FRCP(Edin)
Clinical Director, Neonatal Unit
Simpson Memorial Maternity Pavilion, Edinburgh
and
Senior Lecturer, Department of Child Life and Health
University of Edinburgh

Neil McIntosh
FRCP(Edin), FRCP(Eng)
Professor of Child Life and Health
University of Edinburgh
and
Consultant Paediatrician, Royal Hospital for Sick Children
and Simpson Memorial Maternity Pavilion, Edinburgh

BAILLIÈRE TINDALL
London Philadelphia Toronto Sydney Tokyo

| Baillière Tindall | 24–28 Oval Road, |
| W. B. Saunders | London NW1 7DX |

The Curtis Center,
Independence Square West,
Philadelphia, PA 19106–3399, USA

Harcourt Brace & Company
55 Horner Avenue,
Toronto, Ontario M8Z 4X6, Canada

Harcourt Brace & Company, Australia
  (Pty) Ltd,
30–52 Smidmore Street,
Marrickville, NSW 2204, Australia

Harcourt Brace & Company, Japan
Ichibancho Central Building,
22–1 Ichibancho,
Chiyoda-ku, Tokyo 102, Japan

Typesetting by Fakenham Photosetting Ltd., Fakenham,
Norfolk
Printed by Mackays of Chatham, Chatham, Kent

ISBN 0–7020–1809–0

A catalogue record for this book is available from the British
Library.

Contents

Acknowledgement

The illustrations were drawn by Lesley Skeates Bailey, Medical Artist, Royal Hospital for Sick Children, Edinburgh, UK.

PUBLISHER'S NOTE

Every effort has been made to ensure any dosage recommendations are precise and in agreement with standards officially accepted at the time of publication. However it is urged that you check the manufacturers' recommendations for dosage.

Preface

This handbook is designed as a rapid guide for the medical student and house officer who want to ensure that the maximum information has been obtained during a first consultation. On the evening prior to paediatric undergraduate or postgraduate examinations this handbook provides a system of rapid revision for the 'long case' and 'short case'. To our surprise the postgraduates attending the School of Community Paediatrics have clamoured for the draft to be published, and it is also to be hoped that general practitioners who today take increasing responsibility for community care of the child will find this short volume valuable.

This textbook does not cover any area of *therapy*, but concentrates on all aspects of the interactions between child, doctor and family. We thank all colleagues, medical students and particularly our patients who have taught us much of what follows.

Ian A. Laing
Neil McIntosh

1   The History

HISTORY

Introduction

Hospital is very often a new and worrying environment for parents and children. Allow for this and for limitation in their vocabulary of illness. The child has few if any standards against which to measure their new experience. The history should be received and not extracted. Good eye-to-eye contact with child and parent will build trust rapidly. Do not wear a white laboratory coat. Do not use 'it' when referring to any child, and do not get the gender wrong. Shake hands with both parent and child. Say 'what do you like to be called?' Note down the following details:

Date:
Witness (relationship to child):
Child's name:
> **age:**
> **sex:**
> **race** (can be relevant, e.g. in haemolytic anaemias):

Presenting complaint

1. Allow parents to tell the story in their own words. 'Tell me about . . . '. 'When was . . . last well?'
2. Practise making *aides-mémoires* while looking at the witness's eyes. It is important to look really interested and not just to sound it.
3. Listen intently.
4. Be aware, also, of the child at this stage: activity, sounds, expressions, interest.
5. Then expand the story by cautious questioning based on what the initial remarks suggest. 'Which came first?' It is often helpful to ask questions about comparison with friends and classmates of the same age. You may need to ask about time of onset, site, duration, frequency, relieving factors, exacerbating factors, and any associated features.

SYSTEMATIC ENQUIRY

Central nervous system

- Change in activity or mood, posture, walk, or co-ordination
- Floppiness
- Any alteration of vision
- Onset of headaches (see under 'Pain' below)
- Sleep pattern change
- 'Fits' must be described in great detail, including the time of the episode, tonic and clonic components, the place, the frequency, any triggers (including temper, breath-holding or temperature), associated colour change, incontinence
- Dizziness or faints.

Alimentary system

- Appetite, feeding pattern, evidence of weight loss
- Vomiting (including estimated amount, frequency, timing, nature, stained with blood or bile? Is vomiting effortless or projectile?)
- Constipation (is stool brick-like or just infrequent?)
- Diarrhoea (elicit what is meant by diarrhoea,

whether stool is frequent, semiformed, liquid or offensive; is it truly watery?)

- Character of stools (bulk, frequency, colour, mucus, blood)
- Has there been any apparent pain?
- Any excess thirst or change of drinking pattern?
- In infants discuss feeding:
    Bottle or breast?
    How often?
    How long does a feed take?
    Feeding on demand?
    How is bottle prepared?
    What milk?
    What volume?
    Total intake per day?

If there appears to be a feeding problem you may need to ask 'show me'.

Cardiovascular system

- Breathlessness on exertion
- Central cyanosis
- Apathy
- Slow feeding and weight loss (especially in babies).

Respiratory system

- Discharge from eyes, ears or nose
- Sore throat
- Sputum; any haemoptysis?
- Breathlessness, cyanosis, grunting, stridor
- Wheeze: try to elicit any observed precipitating factors including exercise, dust, animals; is it nocturnal?
- Poor feeding
- Fever
- Cough:
    When?
    At night?
    On exercise?
    Paroxysmal?
    Productive?
    Brassy?

Haemopoietic system

- Pallor
- Listlessness
- Breathlessness
- Bleeding
- Bruising
- Lumps.

Genito-urinary system

- Increased urinary frequency, pain on micturition, force and continuity of urinary stream, loin pain, character of urine (including unusual smell or colour), change in urinary habit
- Late onset enuresis:
    When did bed-wetting begin?
    How often?
    By day?
    Does he/she wake when wet?
    Nappies?
    Toilets?
    Lighting?
    Any dry nights?
    What have you tried so far?
        Restricted fluids?
        Lifting child last thing at night?
    Sibling history?
    Parent history?

Endocrine system

- Growth: need for new clothes and shoes, general build (getting stouter or slimmer)
- Headaches
- Abnormal thirst and urine volumes

- Breast or genital changes (see Figure 2.5)
- Document apathy or change of vision.

Skin

- New marks or spots, eczema, superficial lumps
- Remember any rash can be described in terms of colour, size, feel, distribution, symmetry and the presence of associated features such as weeping, pus or pruritus.

Pain

- When does it occur?
- How long has he/she had it?
- Can you describe it?
- What brings it on?
- Does anything relieve it?
- How long does it last?
- What is its pattern?
- What is its periodicity?
- Are there associated symptoms?
- What does he/she do when it occurs?
- What have you done about it?
- Where is it? Show me. Do you cry?

PAST HISTORY

- Mother's health during pregnancy
- Place of child's birth
- Gestational age at birth
- Mode of delivery
- Birth weight
- Problems around time of birth
- Breast or bottle fed
- Achievement of developmental milestones
- Previous illnesses in chronological order
- Previous hospital admissions, including operations
- Infectious disease contacts
- Details of immunisations
- Allergies and drug hypersensitivities
- Pets at home and their health
- Travel
- Drugs: list all medicines recently taken including dosage, frequency and duration. Establish any drugs already prescribed for the current presenting illness.

If the child has been in a hospital elsewhere and it is probable that the previous notes might prove important, check that there has been no change of name since then. Send for a copy of the previous paediatric notes. Consider also checking the pregnancy and perinatal history from the maternity unit notes.

FAMILY HISTORY

A convenient code system is as in Figure 1.1.

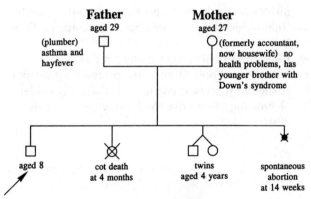

Figure 1.1   Brief family tree

Set out the table from left to right in chronological order. The large arrow indicates the presenting child. Remember consanguinity may be relevant to recessively inherited conditions and is much commoner in certain racial and religious groups.

SOCIAL HISTORY

- Type of house/flat, including number of rooms, number of occupants (including relatives and lodgers), nature of heating, existence of damp
- Any local harassment. Parents employed or not. Financial problems. Tactful questions may elicit a history of single parenthood, significant supportive friends, alcoholism, drug abuse, difficulties with the law
- Cigarette smokers: how many per day?
- Name of school. Is child happy there? Are there particular friends or enemies? Is there any evidence of bullying? Does the child enjoy games or studies best?

2   Examination

INTRODUCTION

The undergraduate and postgraduate should seize every opportunity to examine children. It is essential to develop a confident ease which transmits itself to the parents, to a consultant during professional examinations, and (most important of all) to the child. Once a thorough system becomes completely familiar, the maximum information can be obtained gently and efficiently with the minimum of upset. It *should* be fun.

Preliminary guidelines

1. If possible, avoid having children separated from parents, forcibly undressed and measured. All of these are threats and may make subsequent examination much more difficult. It is not always possible, however, and there may sometimes be merit in having urine specimens obtained and tested before the child is seen by the doctor. Much depends on the sensitivity of the reception staff. Always protect the child's dignity.

2. Never rush into an examination and never place a child flat on a couch or bed without careful preparation. Unless the condition is very acute, quiet friendly contact is time well spent.

3. Make sure the room and your hands are warm. Keep the number of people in the room low. Remember how frightening a crowd of strangers may be.

4. Always talk to the child before touching. Try to keep on the same level physically and in the words and tone used. Talk about toys, clothes, other siblings, friends at school until many of the child's fears are overcome.

5. Start the examination by gently holding and looking at the child's hands. Continue to talk quietly and gently throughout the examination. It may be preferable to examine a partly clothed child, provided all the body is seen step by step. Use blankets to cover legs while the chest is being examined. Cover the trunk while external genitalia are being inspected.

6. Sensitive children may best be examined initially on a parent's knee until they become more confident. With frightened or unco-operative children be opportunist in examining whatever part is offered or available. Improvise and give an infant something to hold as a temporary distraction.

7. Leave uncomfortable procedures (e.g. otoscopy,

pharyngeal inspection, rectal examination) to the end.

8. Give the child some choice, for example, do not ask 'Can I look in your ears?' which invites the answer 'No'. Ask rather 'Which ear would you like me to look in first?'

9. Above all be aware of the child's response to you.

INSPECTION AND GENERAL ASSESSMENT

Paediatric examination begins as the child enters the room. Document dysmorphic features, any unusual gait and inappropriate behaviour.

A child asleep in a parent's arms is a rare luxury: do not wake nor move him/her. Study the breathing pattern, feel the anterior fontanelle, slip a warm stethoscope below the clothes to auscultate the heart, and gently palpate the abdomen for enlargement of the organs or the occurrence of other masses.

Height, weight and head circumference are plotted on appropriate centile charts. The state of hydration can be assessed from the anterior fontanelle in infants, and from the eyes, mouth, skin and, over time, measuring the urine volume and osmolality. Table 2.1 shows the loss of body weight on dehydration.

Table 2.1 Percentage body weight loss on dehydration

Dehydration	Approximate % body weight loss
Mild	5
Moderate	10
Severe	15

Skin

If there is a rash, describe distribution, colour and whether macular, papular, maculopapular, vesicular, bullous, pustular or petechial. Seborrhoea?

Mucous membranes

Mucous membranes are inspected as a very approximate estimate of haemoglobin level.

State of nutrition

Look at axillae, abdomen and thighs, especially for loose skin and creasing with 'skin suit too big for child'.

Pulse

Age	N. range
0-2	80 -140/min
2 - 6	75 - 120/min
> 6	70 - 110/min

Temperature

Document in degrees celsius and add the site, e.g. rectal, axillary, sublingual.

Blood pressure

Blood pressure is taken using an appropriate cuff (i.e. the width of the cuff should cover two-thirds of the distance from shoulder to elbow).

Cardiovascular examination

Inspect for central cyanosis (tongue and inside lips), finger-clubbing and toe-clubbing, and record any tachycardia or tachypnoea.

Palpate both radial pulses and record any disorders of rhythm. Pulse full or low volume. Feel both femoral pulses, and look for old operation scars of patients born with cyanotic heart disease. Palpate the right radial and right femoral pulses together—delay and low volume of the femoral pulse may indicate coarctation of the aorta (Figure 2.1). Look carefully for apex position, and record any chest deformity. Use the palm of the hand to locate a precordial heave or thrill.

Auscultate at the apex to identify the heart sounds— you may need to feel the carotid pulse simultaneously to be sure of the timing. Always listen at the apex, left lower sternal edge, right lower sternal edge, right upper and then left upper sternal edge, left infraclavicular area, the right anterior axillary line, and posteriorly

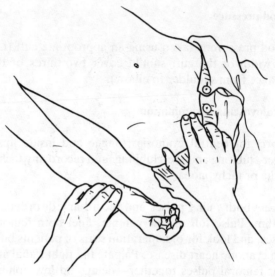

Figure 2.1   Radiofemoral delay

especially just to the left of the vertebral column
(Figure 2.2). If dextrocardia is suspected on clinical
examination, ask the question 'Is it really so or has the
apex been displaced by left pressure or right traction?'

Signs of cardiac failure: tachypnoea, dyspnoea with
feeding, sweating, tachycardia, gallop rhythm, hepatomegaly, unexpected weight gain, crepitations of pul-
monary oedema, cyanosis.

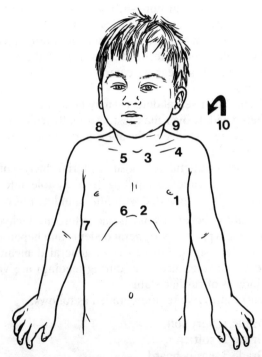

Figure 2.2 Auscultation positions. Recommended order of auscultation: 1, apex; 2, left lower sternal edge; 3, left upper sternal edge; 4, left infraclavicular; 5, right upper sternal edge; 6, right lower sternal edge; 7, right mid-axillary line; 8, right side of neck, 9, left side of neck; 10, posteriorly

Examples of commonly heard murmurs are:

1. Benign flow murmur—heard locally, often at the apex only and may be musical and mid-systolic.
2. Venous hum—heard in the neck and infraclavicular region, but alters with position of the patient and may disappear on compression of the jugular veins.
3. Ventricular septal defect—may be loud, harsh and heard widely over the chest, especially from the left lower sternal edge to the apex, and filling the whole of systole.
4. Persistent ductus arteriosus (arterial duct)—often a musical cadence, spilling from systole into diastole, and associated with full bounding pulses.

Note that the best signs of cardiac failure are tachycardia and tachypnoea: peripheral oedema and hepatomegaly are late signs. Growth rate, general demeanour and exercise tolerance (e.g. during feeding) are valuable indices of cardiac status.

Heart murmurs are often graded as follows:

- Grade 1, very soft
- Grade 2, soft
- Grade 3, easily heard
- Grade 4, easily heard plus a thrill
- Grade 5, very loud plus a thrill: may be audible with the stethoscope above the skin
- Grade 6, audible without a stethoscope

Respiratory examination

Inspect for central cyanosis and finger/toe-clubbing. Record rate of respiration. Are accessory muscles of respiration being used? Record nostril flaring. Describe the chest shape including pigeon chest, hyperinflation, Harrisons's sulci, sternal recession, pectus excavatum. Is indrawing present? Where? If mouth-breathing check the patency of the nares.

Listen—especially for the predominantly inspiratory sound (stridor) of croup, or the prolonged expiratory wheeze of asthma. Remember a sick asthmatic may not wheeze because the tidal volume has been reduced so much: if so this is an EMERGENCY.

Careful percussion, comparing opposite sides of the chest *may* occasionally identify extensive consolidation or effusion, and may confirm the hyper-resonance on the side of a pneumothorax. There is local stony dullness with a pleural effusion or empyema.

Auscultation: Are breath sounds heard equally bilaterally? Rhonchi? Where? What pitch? What phase of respiration? Crepitations? Where? What quality? When? Altering with coughing?

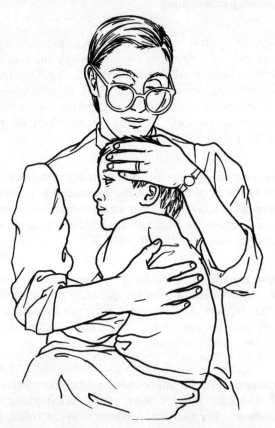

Figure 2.3   Child being held steady for auroscopy

It is often helpful to leave the following part of the examination until last *but it is essential not to forget it.*

Palpate the whole neck and occiput for masses, especially for enlarged lymph nodes. Is there a goitre? Look closely at both ear drums (Figure 2.3), if necessary syringing gently to remove obscuring wax—having first softened the wax with five drops of cerumol 10 min before.

Obtain a brief but adequate view of the oropharynx. For younger children this is often best done on a parent's knee. If a spatula should prove necessary, then a mother's hand firmly on the forehead may help while the child's hands are restrained by her other arm. Note the appearance of the buccal mucosae, gums and dentition.

Abdominal examination

Inspect for distension, movement with respiration, visible peristalsis, skin laxity or dryness, or any superficial abnormalities, e.g. umbilical hernia.

Palpate the abdomen gently with warm hands (Figure 2.4) and using the whole of the flat of the hand. At no time is reassuring talk more important than now, and if possible keep parents close to the child. Watch the child's face closely for apprehension or reaction to pain, particularly as deep palpation begins, no matter

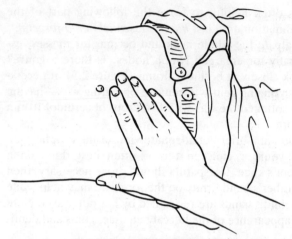

Figure 2.4   Abdominal palpation

how gently. Crying children relax the abdomen briefly during inspiration, allowing a fraction of a second to obtain information. Palpate with gentle fingertips for the liver (1 cm below the right costal margin may be normal), the spleen (which tends to enlarge down the left flank particularly in younger children) and both kidneys (which are often felt in slim co-operative children). Record local tenderness, guarding, or the size, position and quality of any mass. This is often best done by a simple diagram of the child's abdomen.

Percuss for a distended bladder.

Auscultate the bowel sounds.

Rectal examination if indicated is performed with the fifth finger in small children.

Genitalia

Female: labial adhesions, enlargment of the clitoris (e.g. adrenogenital syndrome), perineal excoriation, vaginal discharge.

Male: size and shape of penis, hypospadias +/− chordee, balanitis, position of testes, inguinal hernia (reducible?), hydrocoele (check transillumination to differentiate from haematocoele).

Pubertal Development Grading

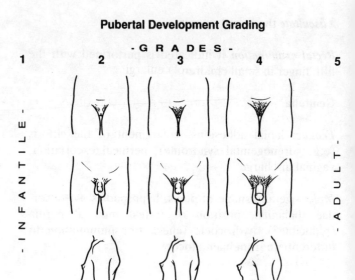

Figure 2.5 Pubertal developmental grading. The top two rows show female and male external genitalia, the bottom row shows breast development.

Pubertal developmental grading

Stages 1 and 5 are fully infantile and fully adult, respectively. You need remember, therefore, only stages 2, 3, and 4 (Figure 2.5).

1. Girls: breast development
    Stage 1: as in early childhood
    Stage 2: breast bud
    Stage 3: breast and areola enlarging
    Stage 4: areola and papilla form a secondary
             mound distinct from enlarging breast
    Stage 5: mature

2. Boys: genital development
    Stage 1: testes, scrotum and penis as in early child-
             hood
    Stage 2: some enlargement of testes and scrotum
    Stage 3: early lengthening of penis
    Stage 4: enlarged penis in length and breadth, with
             glans development
    Stage 5: adult genitalia.

3. Girls and boys: pubic hair
    Stage 1: no pubic hair
    Stage 2: sparse growth of pubic hair each side of
             penile root or on labia
    Stage 3: darker coarse hair meeting on symphysis
    Stage 4: adult hair, no spread to medial surface of
             thighs
    Stage 5: adult in quantity and type with spread to
             medial surface of thighs.

Central nervous system examination

Observe closely the child's alertness, willingness to play, happiness, irritability. With an unconscious child record response to stimuli (e.g. light touch, firm stroke to the skin, shining of bright light). Write down examples of the child's capabilities (e.g. pursues ball under table, plays peek-a-boo, imitates car engine, enjoys make believe, talks articulately ('Mummy, look at the doll').

Record apparent asymmetry, unsteadiness while walking/running/sitting, or any inco-ordination when reaching for toys. Is the gait abnormal? Are there abnormal added movements, jerks, athetoid writhing movements, salaam attacks, episodes of blankness or unusual postures?

Sensation this is often difficult to test reliably and consistently in younger children.

Tone: floppiness. Muscle wasting or fasciculation. Hypertonia, localised (e.g. adductor spasm of the thighs in scissoring of spastic diplegia) or generalised. Any associated clonus.

Power: this is often best done informally by watching a child kick a football or lift a box of bricks. More formally it may be necessary to document systematically power of neck, trunk and limbs, comparing left with right.

Reflexes: jaw, biceps, supinator, triceps, knee, ankle, plantar.

Cranial nerves: remember optic atrophy, strabismus and palatal weakness may be caused either by local defects or as part of the spectrum of cerebral palsy.

See also summary of development in Chapter 5.

3 Neonatal History

INTRODUCTION

Many of the same principles described in Chapters 1 and 2 apply to history-taking and examination of the newborn. A careful account of the problem should be obtained from parents and/or nurse, including an appropriate systematic enquiry—change in urinary habit is not readily identified in a nappied infant, but increased irritability may be an important feature. The following guidelines expand on those already given for older children. In practice much of the information must be gleaned from maternal obstetric notes. The following should be recorded:

Date:
Name:
Date of birth:
Race:
Place of birth:
Presenting history (as in Chapter 1):

Maternal history
- Age
- Parity, and outcome of previous pregnancies
- Previous infertility
- Rubella status
- Health during this pregnancy:
  diabetes, urinary tract infections, hypertension, proteinuria
- Suspicion of large for dates or small for dates
- Ultrasound scan assessments of fetus
- Uterine anomaly
- Complications of pregnancy:
  vaginal bleeding, infections, hydramnios, oligohydramnios
- Drugs taken during pregnancy including alcohol and cigarettes.

Labour and delivery
- Onset of labour, spontaneous?; induced?
- Timing of rupture of membranes and abnormalities of liquor
- Presenting part
- Duration of first and second stage (minutes)
- Mode of delivery, e.g. midcavity forceps with indication
- Problems during labour (e.g. meconium staining of liquor, cord round neck, fetal heart decelerations, type)?

Infant
- Sex
- Birth weight
- Resuscitation: cried immediately at birth? Taken away for treatment (e.g. oxygen)? Drugs given, Apgar scores at 1 and 5 min, any recorded observations (e.g. jitteriness, non-recording dextrostix/BMstix, hypothermia, grunting)?

Placenta
Weight is normally one-fifth to one-sixth of infant's. Cord vessels usually consist of two arteries and one vein.
- Calcification?
- Infarcts?
- Retroplacental clot?
- If twin pregnancy, monochorionic or dichorionic?

4 Neonatal Examination

INTRODUCTION

Examination of the neonate must be carried out in a
warm room free from draughts. Avoid handling infants
immediately before or after a feed. *Talk to the infant*:
the content of what you say may not be critical to the
neonate, but your voice will soothe both child and
parents.

Inspection

- Posture, activity. Describe what you see, for
  example, 'Lying in cot with all four limbs markedly
  flexed' (a hypotonic infant may adopt a frog-like
  posture with both hips abducted)
- An estimate of gestational age may be obtained
  either by experienced observation, or else by the
  use of a Dubowitz chart
- Lethargy or irritability. Quality of cry
- Describe abnormalities seen—polydactyly, spina
  bifida, Down's syndrome

- Record weight, crown–heel length and occipito-frontal circumference on centile chart
- If growth impairment is identified, record crown rump–length also.

Skin

- Colour (jaundiced, pale, plethoric)
- Texture (dry, crinkled, vernix-covered)
- Look for milia, erythema toxicum, haemangiomata (capillary or strawberry?), Mongolian blue spot (usually over lumbrosacral or buttock area) and fat necrosis (hard subcutaneous plaques, especially at a region of previous trauma e.g. forceps blades).

Head

- Describe shape according to Appendix I (see also illustrations in Forfar and Arneil's *Textbook of Paediatrics*, 4th edn, p. 23)
- Fontanelles (bulging or sunken?)
- Feel all sutures and describe over-riding, 'synostosis' (bone fusion)
- Skull bones 'craniotabes' (thinning and softening)
- Moulding, caput succedaneum, cephalhaematoma
- Encephalocoele?

Eyes

Look for discharge of pus or cataract. Increased size, firmness and haziness of the iris may be due to congenital glaucoma. Look for a defect in the iris (coloboma).

Nose

Check for patency of the nares separately, by occluding each in turn while the mouth is closed.

Mouth

Look for thrush on tongue and buccal mucosa, movement of the pharynx, epithelial pearls on the hard palate, cleft lip and/or palate. Describe palatal arch (high, normal, flat) and ranula (mucous cyst on floor of mouth). Look for small mandible (micrognathia).

Spine

Examine whole of midline posteriorly for hairy patch, dimple, naevus or cyst. Palpate the entire spine. Is there scoliosis or kyphosis? Beware aplasia of the lumbosacral area in infants of diabetic mothers.

Limbs

Count fingers and toes, examine palmar creases and look for positional deformities. Varus or valgus deformities of the ankle should be differentiated as to whether they are fully correctable by passive manipulation. Examine hips with Ortolani's test (Figure 4.1).

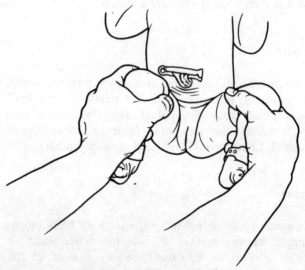

Figure 4.1   Hip examination

Central nervous system

- Posture, tone
- Primitive reflexes: root, suck, swallow, grasp, step, place, Moro, tonic neck. Rotate upright infant for labyrinthine control of eye movements and opto-kinetic nystagmus
- Vision: screws up eyes to light
- Assess head control with *gentle* pull to sit (Figure 4.2)

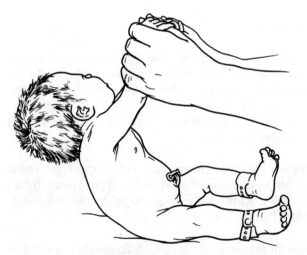

Figure 4.2   Pull to sit

- Phasic reflexes: biceps, knee, ankle and toe. Also test for clonus
- N.B. 'Hemisyndrome' refers to any unilateral abnormality of neurological signs
- Palsies
  (a) Facial, common, usually gone in 48 h
  (b) Erb's—traction injury, arm extended and medially rotated, usually resolved in 2 weeks
  (c) Klumpke's—less common, claw hand and absent grasp. Look for associated Horner's syndrome.

Abdomen

Observe any distension (the newborn's abdomen is often protuberant), beware the taut, drum-like distension which may signify obstruction. The abdomen may be scaphoid in dehydration or in high atresia and especially in diaphragmatic hernia. Peristalsis. Inspect for umbilical hernia.

Palpate the liver (often 1 cm below the right costal margin in the normal newborn) and the spleen (often tippable). Kidneys are frequently palpable and ballottable (Figure 4.3).

Feel for inguinal hernias, and differentiate from hydrocoele. Transilluminate the scrotum to differentiate

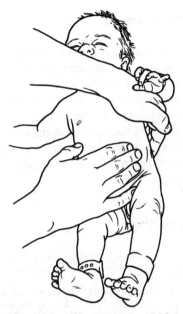

Figure 4.3 Palpating spleen/kidney

hydrocoele from haematocoele. Examine anus for
patency: has meconium been passed? Look carefully at
genitalia: the labia may be completely or partially
fused. Is the clitoris enlarged? Are testes in the scrotum
aberrant or undescended. Position of urethral meatus:
hypospadias? Epispadias? Is it glandular, and is there
hooding of the prepuce as in chordee?

Cardiovascular system

See pages 15–18, but note that in the neonatal period the murmur of the ductus arteriosus is common, is usually temporary and may be confined to systole. The finding of femoral pulses in the early days of life does not exclude a coarctation of the aorta.

Note that causes of tachypnoea in the newborn are as follows: hunger, overheating, cold, discomfort, birth asphyxia, anaemia, cardiac failure, respiratory disease, metabolic disease.

FURTHER READING

Dubowitz L.M.S., Dubowitz V. and Goldberg C. (1970) Clinical assessment of gestational age in the newborn infant. *Journal of Pediatrics* **77**: 1–10.

Forfar J.O. History taking, physical examination and screening. In: (A.G.M. Campbell and N. McIntosh, eds) *Forfar and Arneil's Textbook of Paediatrics* 4th Edn (1992). Churchill Livingstone.

5 Summary of Development

INTRODUCTION

There are several long and detailed volumes written about childhood development. However, the *rapid* summary here will give a paediatrician a reliable guide to the developmental milestones most commonly seen. *Beware* the great variation in developmental achievement. It may be normal for a child to walk precociously at 10 months, or to take the first faltering steps at 20 months. Only by extensive experience can a practitioner separate the normal from the abnormal. It is critical that the paediatrician becomes familiar with a system of examination, and practises it frequently. Only then can subtle abnormalities be detected and normal variations be explained confidently to the anxious parent.

Newborn

- Can suck, swallow, cry, hear and respond to light
- Reflexes include root, suck, grasp, pull to sit (with marked head lag), doll's eye and (after a few days) optokinetic nystagmus, stepping, placing, Moro (Figure 5.1) and tonic neck reflex (Figure 5.2)

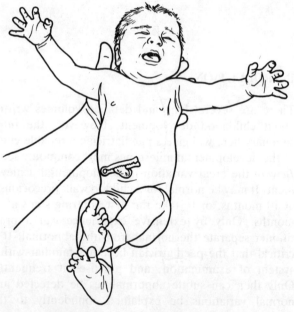

Figure 5.1 Moro reflex in newborn

• Note that the reflexes when elicited in the order given above can be done in a smooth sequence lifting the infant only once.

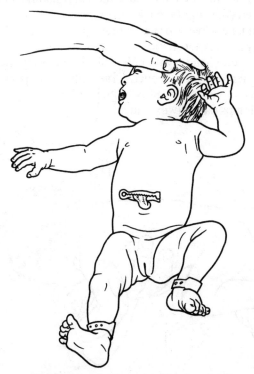

Figure 5.2   Tonic neck reflex in newborn

Six weeks

- Supine lies with head to one side, with the ipsilateral limbs extended and the contralateral limbs flexed (fencing stance posture)
- Can fix, follow and may smile
- May coo responsively
- Moderate head lag on pull to sit. Prone brings head momentarily off couch. In ventral suspension (Figure 5.3) the head is in line with the body, and with hips partially extended.

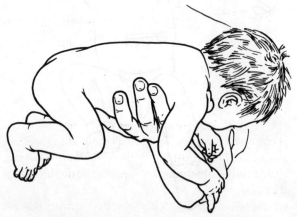

Figure 5.3   Ventral suspension in 6 week old

Three months

- Supine, lies with head in the midline
- Hands loosely open. Has hand regard and may show early finger play (Figure 5.4)

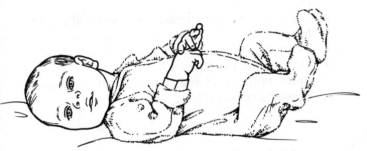

Figure 5.4   Supine finger play in 3 month old

- On ventral suspension brings head momentarily above level of back. Prone brings head and upper chest off couch. Little or no head lag on pull to sit
- Excites with appearance of feeding bottle if hungry
- Babbles
- Quietens to sound of rattle of spoon in cup. Inhibiting primitive reflexes.

Six months

- Supine, lifts head off couch to look at feet, lifts leg and grasps foot
- Reaches for toys with palmar grasp
- Regards rolling ball at 2–3 metres (approx. 5–10 feet)
- Transfers object from hand to mouth and hand to hand
- May tripod-sit
- May roll front to back
- Prone brings head and chest high off couch on to extended elbows (Figure 5.5)

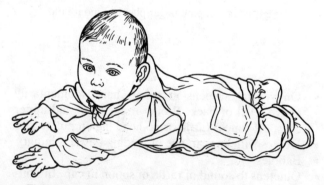

Figure 5.5 Prone, with arms extended, in 6 month old

- Downward parachute (Figure 5.6) readily seen
- Laughs, squeals, is visually insatiable
- Accurately turns to low intensity rattle at ear level within 0.5 metres (approx. 18 inches) (Figure 5.7)
- Puts hands to bottle and pats it when feeding.

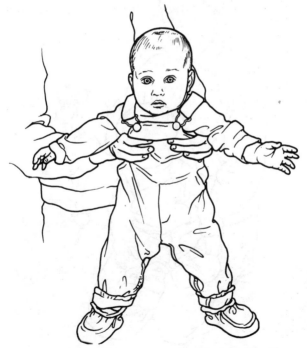

Figure 5.6 Downward parachute in 6 month old

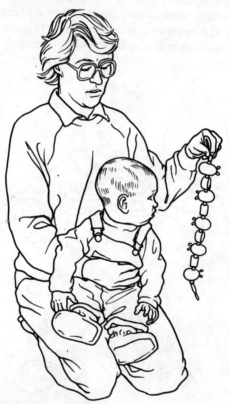

Figure 5.7   Turns to soft sound, 6 months old

Nine months

- Stable while sitting for 10 min on floor, and can pick up toy without overbalancing
- Rolls. Beginning to crawl or squirm
- Pulls to stand, but falls back with a bump

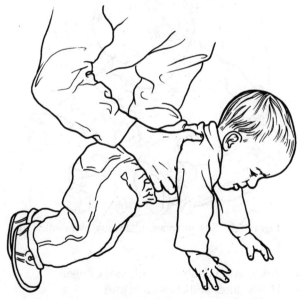

Figure 5.8   Forward parachute, 9 months old

- Claps hands
- Understands 'No' and 'Bye bye'
- Forward parachute reflex present (Figure 5.8)
- Manipulates toys with interest (Figure 5.9)

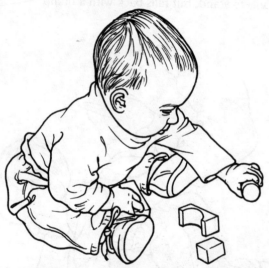

Figure 5.9   Sits and manipulates toys, 9 months old

- Pokes at small objects with index finger
- Holds, bites and chews a biscuit
- Plays peek-a-boo and imitates hand-clapping.

One year

- Pulls to standing
- Cruises round furniture and controls return to floor
- May walk independently
- Helps with dressing

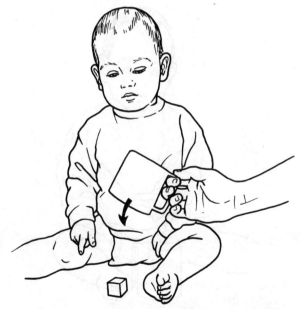

Figure 5.10(a)   Parent concealing toy, 1 year old

- Bilateral neat pincer grasp
- Sometimes gives toys to adults on request
- Throws away deliberately
- Likes pictures
- Looks in correct place for objects which have rolled out of sight
- Finds toy under a cup (Figure 5.10)

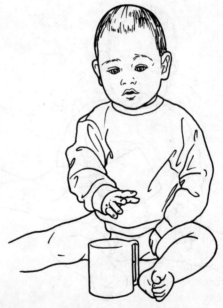

Figure 5.10(b)   One year old reaches for cup

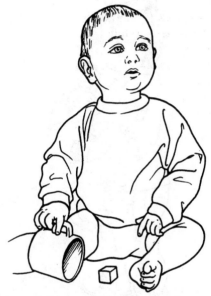

Figure 5.10(c) Finds toy under cup

- Understands several words
- Responds to own name
- May say 'Dada, Mama, Baba'
- Drinks from a cup.

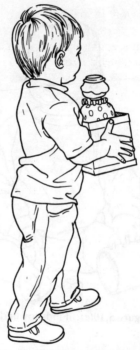

Figure 5.11 Walks alone, 18 months old

Fifteen months

- Walks with uneven broad-based gait
- Crawls upstairs
- Builds tower of two cubes in imitation

- Grasps crayon in palmar grasp and scribbles in imitation
- Has several recognisable words in correct context
- Obeys simple instructions
- Brings spoon to mouth and licks it
- Carries doll by leg, arm or hair.

Eighteen months

- To and fro scribbling with pencil held in palmar grasp at mid shaft
- Builds tower of three cubes in imitation
- Turns book pages and recognises everyday objects
- Enjoys nursery rhymes
- Early singing
- Knows several parts of the body
- Holds spoon and takes food to mouth
- Takes off shoes and socks
- May have bowel control but this is very variable
- Steady purposeful walk (Figure 5.11).

Two years

- Spontaneous circular scribbling with pencil held between thumb and first two fingers. Imitates vertical line, circle and occasionally T and V
- Can walk, run, squat (Figure 5.12) and climb stairs using two feet per step

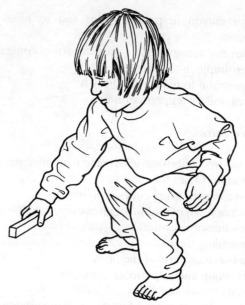

Figure 5.12   Squats to pick up fallen toy, 2 years old

- Imitates parental domestic duties
- Feeds with a spoon without much spilling
- May be dry by day
- Builds tower of six cubes. May have vocabulary of 50 words, and may use three-word sentences

- Joins in nursery rhymes
- Tantrums may be common.

Three years

- Climbs stairs one foot per step
- Pedals a tricycle
- Can run on tiptoe
- Copies a circle and may imitate a cross
- May draw a man with a head and some line representation of the rest of body
- Cuts with scissors
- Speaks in sentences, and may know a few colours, recites nursery rhymes and counts to ten
- During play commonly speaks in a monologue of make-believe
- Eats with fork and spoon
- May be dry through the night (very variable).

Four years

- Walks up and down stairs one foot per step
- May hop
- May wash, dress and undress, but not yet managing to tie laces
- Listens to long stories
- May draw a man with a head, trunk and legs and occasionally with arms and fingers

- Can draw a cross in imitation, holding pencil in adult fashion
- Good grammatical speech but with a few infantilisms
- Counts to twenty or more
- Washes and dries hands
- Enjoys simple jokes.

Five years

- Climbs, slides and swings, skips on alternate feet
- Threads large needles
- Builds three steps from six cubes, and sometimes four steps from ten cubes
- Copies a square and may copy a triangle
- Draws a man with head, trunk, limbs, fingers and some facial features
- Draws a house with door, windows, roof and chimney
- Grammatical speech but may still confuse the 's, f, th' group
- Uses knife and fork
- Dresses and undresses alone.

6 Child Abuse

INTRODUCTION

The subject of child abuse is fraught with difficulties. The given history may be untrue, only partly true, or may be a completely accurate account. The physical examination must be sensitively handled, must be complete, and should be documented in obsessional detail. In practice there should be early involvement by a senior member of staff, especially since there may be future medico-legal implications.

Definitions

1. Neglect (accounts for 60% of child abuse): failure to provide basic shelter, supervision or support, or actively exposing the child to a hazardous situation.
2. Physical abuse (20%): debate about what is acceptable abuse—corporal punishment.
3. Emotional abuse (17%): difficult to define and detect—the wilful destruction or impairment of a child's feeling of competence.

4. Sexual abuse (6%): inappropriate exposure to sexual acts or materials, and passive use of children as sexual stimuli for adults (child pornography).

EVALUATION OF THE HISTORY

1. Any history must be very carefully recorded.
2. Look for improbable or inconsistent stories or stories that change over time.
3. If a child is old enough, get the child's *spontaneous* account (ideally separated from family, but if another family member is present, ensure eye-to-eye contact is *not* possible).
4. Be alert for elements of the history that do not fit with clinical experience or sense (e.g. the young baby with a fractured skull 'from falling off the bed on to a carpeted floor').

REVIEW OF SYSTEMS

Are there feeding difficulties such as colic, food refusal or difficulties in toilet training? **Are the** parents expecting too much too soon from their baby or child? Is the child being difficult and wilful? **Are there** behaviour problems, especially of recent onset (e.g. running away, deterioration in schoolwork, violent behaviour, withdrawal, enuresis or encopresis)?

THE UNSPOKEN HISTORY

Parents sometimes do not tell the truth!

1. This may be because, as in the syndrome of child abuse, they feel guilty about something they have done or have omitted to do. They may want reassurance that they have not injured their child badly. Sometimes they may be indicating that they wish for personal and even psychiatric help.

2. Alternatively it may be that the parents are at their wit's end and wish for help. They think it unlikely that the doctor will be sympathetic simply about their anxiety so they invent symptoms or problems (e.g. constipation, diarrhoea, vomiting, not feeding, always crying, never sleeping) so that the doctor has to take them and their child seriously. In this situation it is very important not to be superior and dismissive of the voiced complaints, but to accept that there is a significant underlying problem of some sort (usually in the parent), for example, a fear that if the child does not stop crying they may lose control and hit out. Acknowledge their worries: 'You must be very worried about that Mrs Smith, is it getting you down? Do you think we might help by admitting John for a few days to see what's going on?' This takes the strain off the mother and father and allows you time to get information from the general prac-

titioner, nursery, social workers, etc, as to whether there are social problems, or other difficulties that can be rectified.

3. The parents may also be causing fictitious illness or real illness or injury to their child to get attention that they themselves require emotionally (Munchausen's syndrome by proxy). Classically the mother is a model mother, always being very helpful on the ward.

EXAMINATION

This should be done in good light with a ruler and anatomical diagrams. Photographs should be taken as soon as possible after the complete examination and should be repeated several days later when bruises may be more obvious. Both written descriptions and diagrams should be as accurate as possible. Note lack of clean clothing and poor personal hygiene of parent or child. Does the child separate too easily from the parents? Is he/she excessively fearful, withdrawn, unresponsive, angry or destructive?

1. *Bruises*: normal over bony areas such as shins, elbows and forehead, but not on soft areas, particularly inside of arms (when child defends head and face). Bilateral injuries to the face are unlikely

to be natural. Bruises at first are red/purple: Look at shape—belt buckle or hand slap? Differential diagnosis: Mongolian blue spots, thrombocytopenia, meningococcal disease, Henoch–Schoenlein purpura, sensitivity vasculitis, haemophilia, folk medicine practices (cupping). With significant bruising, do a platelet count and clotting screen.

2. *Bites*: semicircular or crescent shaped. They may or may not break the skin. Measure and photograph. They darken with time, so a second photograph may be warranted.

3. *Burns*: measure shape, extent and depth. Is there a glove and stocking distribution (from immersion in hot water)? Is there the shape of a hot object (e.g. cigarette or hair curlers)? Inflicted burns are rarely first degree.

4. *Head injuries*: are there signs of injury (e.g. depressed fracture or a bulging fontanelle)? Are the sutures split? Is there hair loss? Look for bruising over the mastoid (Battle's sign), black eyes (racoon eyes) or blood behind the ear drum indicating a basilar fracture.

5. *Eyes*: dilate the pupils—are there retinal haemorrhages, indicating possibly a shaking injury, blows to the head or chest compression?

6. *Abdominal injuries*: duodenal haematoma present as abdominal pain, anorexia and retroperitoneal mass. Beware ruptured bowel, stomach or spleen.

7. ***Genitalia***: *Note that most sexually abused children have completely normal genitalia.*
   Female: prepubertal girls usually have a small amount of clear non-odorous discharge. Exceptions to this are the neonate in the first week, and 6 months or so prior to menarche when the discharge may be thicker and grey-white. Discharge may be from sexually transmitted diseases, foreign bodies, poor hygiene and irritants such as bubble baths. Inspection of the introitus and a rectal examination to feel anteriorly are important, and any bruises, lacerations, irritation, bleeding, warts or erythematous papules should be noted. An otoscope may allow magnification, retracting the labia minora until the hymen is visible. Check the size of the opening (normally less than 6 mm) and for bruising, bleeding or scarring.
   Male: look for bruising, erythema or discharge from the penis.

8. ***Rectum***: haemorrhoids or skin tags (other than the midline anteriorly) are suspicious. The anal dilation reflex is not pathognomonic of penetration but may be present quite commonly. It is also found in severe constipation and sometimes in normal children.

9. ***Skeletal trauma***: Bony injuries are most common in abused infants less than 3 years of age. A full skeletal survey should be done. X-rays may need to be

repeated. Fractures of different ages suggest injury on more than one occasion. The differential diagnosis includes congenital syphilis, scurvy, infantile cortical hyperostosis, osteogenesis imperfecta and Menkes' kinky hair syndrome and rarely, leukaemia, neuroblastoma and osteomyelitis.

Laboratory evidence of sexual abuse: 25% of sexually abused children may have sexually transmitted diseases at the time of the initial examination. *Gonococcus*, *Chlamydia*, *Trichomonas*, condylomata acuminata (papillomavirus) and genital warts are probably pathognomonic of sexual abuse. Although perinatal transmission of the last can occur, nevertheless, over the first year of life, only laryngeal papillomata are known to occur. It is vital that a chain of evidence be maintained for sexually transmitted disease and other specimens associated with childhood assault of any nature—this is a *written* record making certain that the specimen that arrives in the laboratory is the same as that taken from the patient.

7 Passing Professional Examinations

INTRODUCTION

Whether the undergraduate is preparing for professional examinations in paediatrics, or the postgraduate is intent on passing the Diploma in Child Health or the Membership of the Royal College of Physicians, certain principles apply and are frequently forgotten by the unwary. The following brief account should help the candidate to maximise the chance of passing. Remember it is only a rather cruel game.

Equipment

- Stethoscope
- Tape measure
- Auroscope
- Ophthalmoscope
- Rattle

- Ask for centile charts
- Sphygmomanometer
- Toys as appropriate.

Simple rules

1. Dress smartly, look professional.
2. Smile.
3. Don't fight with any of the examiners.
4. Speak clearly, remember that their auditory meati may not be in the first flush of youth.
5. Keep good eye-to-eye contact with your examiner.
6. Introduce yourself to the children and parents.
7. If you suspect you know more about the subject than your examiner, do not embarrass him/her, but rather retreat into a diplomatic solution such as 'This is a controversial area, but a recent leading article in *Archives* has suggested that ... ', then make your point courteously. Be sure a leading article *did* make the point!
8. Remember everyone encounters the screaming child or thoroughly unco-operative patient. Keep your cool. Get as much information as you can without making a permanent enemy of the child, and then tell the examiner that in clinical practice you would normally return to complete the examination at a time more convenient for the patient.

9. In cross-table interviews do not:
    (a) lean in a bored way on the table
    (b) stare out of the window as you think/reply
    (c) offer the examiner a handsome bribe
    (d) be obsequious
    (e) worry if you come to the end of your knowledge on a particular subject, a good examiner will change topic.
10. Do keep it simple. You have only one ambition; that is to pass. Usually this is easier than you suppose. Even the MRCP examination is based on simple principles and involves thoroughness, competence, but very few subtleties.
11. Read the main articles in the leading journals of the last 3 months (e.g. *Archives of Diseases in Childhood*, *The British Medical Journal*, *The Journal of Pediatrics* and *Pediatrics*). Try to predict a few 'hot topics' which might be discussed at interview.
12. Remember that the candidate who shows that he/she handles children well and discusses simply and logically is more likely to pass than the bookworm who knows every last detail about Schimmelpenning–Fuerstein–Mims syndrome.

Appendix I: Description of Head Shapes

Because infants have little scalp hair their head shape is obvious. Moulding from the birth process quickly disappears. A degree of asymmetry (plagiocephaly) is very common and is without implication. Low-birth-weight preterm infants often develop some head-flattening from side to side and compensatory elongation (dolicocephaly). Craniostenosis (fusing of bones) can result in unusual head shapes (e.g. acrocephaly).

Table A.I   Head shapes

Head shape	Description
Microcephalic (small-headed)	Small cranial vault
Megalencephalic (large-headed)	Large cranial vault
Hydrocephalic (water-headed)	Large cranial vault due to enlarged ventricles
Brachycephalic (short-headed)	Short cranial vault from front to back
Dolicocephalic (long-headed)	Elongated skull from front to back
Oxycephalic (sharp-headed)	Long, pointed head
Acrocephalic (top-headed)	Elongated skull with prominent vertex
Turricephalic (tower-headed)	High elongated skull with flat top
Scaphocephalic (keel-shaped)	Long narrow skull often with prominent sagittal ridge
Plagiocephalic (oblique-headed)	Asymmetrical skull

Appendix II: United Kingdom Immunisation Programme

Triple vaccine: Diphtheria, Tetanus, Pertussis

One 0.5 ml dose of a mixture in isotonic buffer solution of diphtheria toxoid and tetanus toxoid adsorbed on to an aluminium hydroxide gel, together with not more than 20 000 million killed *Bordetella pertussis* organisms.

Give three doses—**at 2, 3 and 4 months** irrespective of gestational age.

Dose 0.5 ml deep subcutaneous or intramuscular injection.

Contraindications
- An evolving neurological problem
- Parental refusal despite counselling
- During an acute febrile illness
- Severe local or systemic reaction to a previous dose.

Booster dose of adsorbed diphtheria/tetanus should be

given prior to school entry, at least 3 years after the primary course. A further booster of tetanus alone is recommended at ages 15 to 19, or before leaving school.

Polio

Routinely, this is available as live attenuated virus (containing antigens of Types I, II and III). The dose is 0.5 ml orally **at 2, 3 and 4 months**, given at the same time as the triple vaccine. Also, a booster before school and at ages 15 to 19 or before leaving school. Inactivated polio virus is available for infants in whom attenuated virus may be contraindicated: in immuno-compromised infants (e.g. children with malignant conditions of the reticuloendothelial system, those receiving steroid therapy, siblings of immunocompromised children), a primary course is given as 0.5 ml deep subcutaneous or intramuscular; three doses at monthly intervals from 2 months.

Haemophilus influenzae type B (Hib)

This is a conjugate vaccine, dose 0.5 ml, given **at 2, 3 and 4 months** of life. A course is indicated for children less than 13 months of age who have not previously been vaccinated. Can be given at the same time as the triple vaccine and polio immunisation, or else the course can be completed later.

Measles/Mumps/Rubella (MMR)

A freeze-dried preparation of live attenuated measles, mumps and rubella viruses, dose 0.5 ml, is given deep subcutaneously or intramuscularly. It is recommended that MMR is given to all children of both sexes from **12 to 15 months** of age. It should be given to any child of any age, not previously immunised, and whose parents request it.

Contraindications include an acute febrile illness, immunocompromised children (immunosuppressive therapy, high dose steroids), malignant disease, children who have received another live vaccine (e.g. BCG) in the last 3 weeks, or who have received an immunoglobulin injection in the previous 3 months, or who have had a previous anaphylactic reaction to egg.

Bacille Calmette–Guérin vaccine (BCG)

The freeze-dried vaccine is given intradermally by a 25 or 26 gauge needle and a tuberculin syringe. Inject over the insertion of the deltoid muscle; dose 0.1 ml. Adverse reactions include abscesses, ulcers and keloid formation. A modified Heaf gun may be used in neonates and very young children only. Administer to:

(a) school children aged 10 to 13 years
(b) all students

(c) all children whose parents request it
(d) at risk children; contacts of known cases of active respiratory tuberculosis
(e) children of families whose origin is from the Far East, the Indian subcontinent, Africa, or Central or South America.

Contraindications include: those on steroid or other immunosuppressive therapy, those with malignancies of the reticuloendothelial system, those HIV positive, those pregnant, and those with positive sensitivity tests to tuberculin protein.

Hepatitis B

The vaccine contains $20\,\mu g\,ml^{-1}$ of hepatitis B surface antigen (HBsAg). Dosage for children is 0.5 ml intramuscularly given **at the elected time, then 1 month later and then 6 months after the first dose**. Antibody titres may be checked 2 to 4 months after completion of the course. Those with antibody levels greater than $100\,mi.u.\,ml^{-1}$ have responded, while those with lower levels may require a booster dose, or even a complete new course of vaccination.

The vaccine is recommended for all those whose lifestyle puts them in contact with known cases or carriers. It is contraindicated if the patient is HBsAg positive, or has acute hepatitis B. Risk groups include those with haemophilia or chronic renal failure, health care workers, parenteral drug abusers, those (homosexual or heterosexual) who change sexual partners frequently, close family contacts of a known case or carrier, and babies born of mothers who are chronic hepatitis B carriers or who had acute hepatitis B during pregnancy.

Hepatitis B immunoglobulin (HBIG) provides passive immunity. It is available in 2 ml ampoules containing 200 i.u. or 5 ml ampoules containing 500 i.u. For the newborn at risk 2 ml should be given *as soon as possible after birth*. The dosage is 200 i.u. for children of up to 4 years old, and 300 i.u. for those of 5 to 9 years. The active vaccine and the passive immunoglobulin can, if indicated, be given in separate injections, at different sites but at the same time.

Appendix III: Useful Definitions

PERINATAL

Abortion: product of conception born dead before 24 weeks gestation.

Birth rate: number of births per 1000 population.

Embryo: the human conceptus for the first 10 weeks after conception (and in practice for the first 12 weeks measured from the first day of mother's last menstrual period).

Extreme low birth weight: weighing less than or equal to 1000 g at the time of birth.

Extreme preterm: gestation less than 28 completed weeks measured from the first day of mother's last menstrual period.

Fetus: the human conceptus after the embryonic phase until the moment of delivery.

Hydramnios: excessive amount of amniotic fluid.

Infant mortality rate: number of deaths in the first year of life per 1000 live births.

Low birth weight: weighing less than or equal to 2500 g at the time of birth.

Neonatal mortality rate: number of deaths in the first month of life per 1000 live births.

Oligohydramnios: diminished volume of amniotic fluid.

Perinatal mortality rate: number of stillbirths and first week neonatal deaths per 1000 total births.

Polyhydramnios: excessive amount of amniotic fluid.

Post-term: gestation greater than 42 weeks measured from the first day of mother's last menstrual period.

Preterm: gestation less than 37 completed weeks measured from the first day of mother's last menstrual period.

Small for gestational age: birth weight less than the tenth centile for a given gestation.

Stillbirth: child born dead after 24 weeks gestation.

Term: gestation 37 completed weeks to 42 completed weeks after the first day of mother's last menstrual period.

Very low birth rate: weighing less than or equal to 1500 g at the time of birth.

GROWTH

Failure to thrive: inadequate growth velocity.

Height velocity: centimetres increase in 1 year at that age (quote as centile).

Weight velocity: kilogrammes increase in 1 year at that age (quote as centile).

GENETIC/DYSMORPHOLOGY

Arachnodactyly: long slender (spidery) digits.

Camptodactyly: permanent flexion of an interphalangeal joint, usually of the fifth finger.

Clinodactyly: permanent deflexion of one or more fingers.

Congenital: present at the time of birth.

Consanguinity: related by blood (usually of related parents, e.g. first cousins).

Cryptorchidism: failure of descent of the testes.

Dysmorphism: having unusual physical features (e.g. low set ears, syndactyly).

Glossoptosis: downward displacement of the tongue.

Hypomandibularism: smallness of the mandible.

Micrognathia: smallness of the mandible.

Phocomelia: flipper limb (e.g. seen after thalidomide teratogenesis).

Polydactyly: the presence of more than five digits on a hand or foot.

Ranula: sublingual cyst.

Syndactyly: the joining together of two or more fingers or toes.

Syndrome: a pattern of unusual features (e.g. Down's or cri-du-chat).

Teratogenic: causing embryonic or fetal abnormality.

NEUROLOGICAL

Ataxia: a loss of motor co-ordination.
Athetosis: a condition of constant involuntary slow writhing movements.
Cerebral palsy: a motor disorder resulting from a non-progressive lesion of the developing brain.
Diplegia: a type of cerebral palsy with symmetrical paresis of the limbs, especially the lower limbs, and usually with rigidity or spasticity.
Dysarthria: difficulty co-ordinating speech.
Dysdiadochokinesis: difficulty in performing rapid alternating movements.
Dyskinesia: difficulty with voluntary movement.
Dysmetria: difficulty judging distance.
Hemiparesis: partial paralysis of one side of the body.
Hemiplegia: paralysis of one side of the body.
Myalgia: muscle pain.
Quadriplegia: paralysis affecting all four limbs.
Syncope: fainting.

RESPIRATORY

Dyspnoea: difficulty with breathing.
Hyperpnoea: overbreathing.
Orthopnoea: difficulty with breathing except when erect (either standing or sitting).
Pectus carinatum: pigeon chest (prominent sternum).

Pectus excavatum: hollow chest (sternal depression).

Stridor: a sound, predominantly inspiratory in character, resulting from the rapid passage of air through a partially obstructed larynx or trachea.

Tachypnoea: rapid respiration.

Wheeze: a musical sound, predominantly expiratory in character, resulting from the rapid passage of air through partially obstructed bronchi.

DERMATOLOGICAL

Alopecia: baldness.

Blister: an elevated serum-filled lesion.

Bruise: bleeding into the subcutaneous tissues.

Bulla: a large blister.

Ecchymosis: a purple area caused by extravasation of blood into the skin.

Exanthema: a skin eruption as a symptom of a general disease (e.g. measles).

Haemangioma: a vascular lesion, usually congenital.

Ichthyosis: dry scaly skin.

Impetigo: a pustular skin rash caused by staphylococci or streptococci.

Lentigo: a brown macule like a freckle with a regular border.

Macule: a circumscribed non-palpable discolouration of the skin.

Morbilliform: measles-like.

Naevus: a vascular, pigmented or hairy skin lesion, usually congenital.

Papule: a small raised palpable lesion.

Petechiae: pinhead purpura.

Pruritus: itchiness.

Purpura: multiple spontaneous haemorrhages into skin or mucous membranes.

Pustule: an elevated pus-containing lesion.

Seborrhoea: overaction of the sebaceous glands.

Telangiectasia: localised capillary dilation.

Urticaria (hives, nettle rash): an eruption of itching wheals.

Varicelliform: chickenpox-like.

Verruca: a wart.

Vesicle: a blister 0.5 cm or less in diameter.

Vitiligo: a condition of skin depigmentation.

Wheal: an urticarial eruption: a pink or white raised area surrounded by a flare of erythema.

GENITO-URINARY

Balanitis: inflammation of the foreskin.

Chordee: ventral angulation of the shaft of the penis.

Enuresis: involuntary passage of urine, usually used of bed wetting.

Epispadias: with the urethral orifice emerging on the dorsum of the penis.

Hydrocoele: a collection of serous fluid in the tunica vaginalis of the scrotum.

Hypospadias: with the urethral orifice emerging on the under surface of the penis.

GASTROINTESTINAL

Atresia: congenital absence of an opening, passage or cavity, especially with reference to complete bowel blockage due to failure of development of the lumen.

Bulimia: morbidly increased appetite often alternating with periods of anorexia.

Encopresis: involuntary passage of faeces.

Intussusception: the infolding of one segment of intestine within another.

Scaphoid: hollowed out.

Stenosis: narrowing.

EAR, NOSE AND THROAT

Epistaxis: nose bleeding.

Glue ear: serous otitis media.

VISUAL

Amblyopia: partial loss of sight.

Aniridia: absence of the iris.

Aphakia: absence of the crystalline lens.

Chalazion: a chronic inflammatory granuloma of the eyelid.

Coloboma: a congenital cleft of the iris.

Hordeolum: stye.

Hyphema: blood in anterior chamber of the eye.

Strabismus: a squint.

Uveitis: inflammation of the iris, ciliary body and choroid.

ORTHOPAEDIC

Genu recurvatum: a condition of hyperextension of the knee.

Genu valgum: knock-kneed.

Genu varum: bow-legged.

Gibbus: extreme kyphosis with a sharply angulated segment.

Kyphosis: an abnormal curvature of the spine with convexity backwards.

Osteomyelitis: inflammation of the bone marrow and adjacent bone.

Osteopetrosis: marbling of the bones leading to obliteration of the marrow.

Osteoporosis: diminished mineralisation of bones.

Scoliosis: lateral curvature of the spine.

Talipes calcaneovalgus: club foot with dorsal flexion (i.e. heel on ground) and eversion.

Talipes equinovarus: club foot, with extension and inversion at the ankle.

Appendix IV: Patterns of Cerebral Palsy

Cerebral palsy is the motor manifestation of non-progressive brain damage of varied aetiology, and sustained during the period of brain growth *in utero*, during infancy or during early childhood.

The children may display features in the following *neurophysiological* categories:

(a) **spasticity and rigidity**, indicating damage to the pyramidal tracts;
(b) **dyskinetic movements** indicating damage to extra-pyramidal tracts;
(c) **ataxia**;
(d) **mixed** picture of the above;
(e) rarely persistent **hypotonia**.

Cerebral palsy can also be described *anatomically*:

(a) **Quadriparesis** involving all four limbs;
(b) **Diplegia** involving primarily the lower extremities;
(c) **Hemiparesis** involving one half of the body, usually predominantly the upper limb.

In children with **spastic** type of cerebral palsy hypertonicity of muscles leads to characteristic posture and gait abnormalities and to joint contractures.

Ataxia is important in about 10% of infants with cerebral palsy, and may commonly be due to genetic factors, but occasionally to cerebellar damage or damage to the vertebral arteries during delivery. Clinically the ataxia may manifest as dysmetria, tremor, broad-based gait and dysdiadochokinesis.

Dyskinetic cerebral palsy in the United Kingdom represents a small number, the majority of whom had problems around the time of birth including extreme prematurity, birth asphyxia or severe jaundice. In later childhood the defect presents as choreoathetoid movements, deafness, loss of upward conjugate gaze, dysarthria and poor hand manipulation.

Appendix V: Normal Parameters

Table A.V Pulse, respiration and blood pressure: normal range or mean value at a given age

	Newborn at term	1 year old	10 years old	15 years old
Pulse at rest (beats per minute)	100–140	70–100	75–90	60–80
Respirations at rest (breaths per minute)	30–60	25–40	15–30	12–20
Blood pressure (mm Hg)	80/40	90/45	100/50	115/65

Index